Wendy Lewis

wrinkle rescue

the lowdown on smoothing facial lines

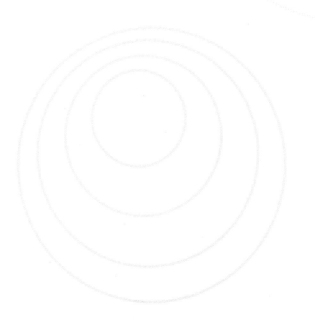

QUADRILLE

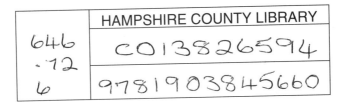
Editorial Director: **Jane O'Shea**

Creative Director: **Mary Evans**

Designer: **Sue Storey**

Project Editor: **Lisa Pendreigh**

Editor: **Katie Ginn**

Picture Research: **Nadine Bazar**

Illustrations: **Sue Storey**

Production: **Nancy Roberts**

First published in 2002 by Quadrille Publishing Limited
Alhambra House
27–31 Charing Cross Road
London WC2H OLS

Printed and bound in Singapore

Contents

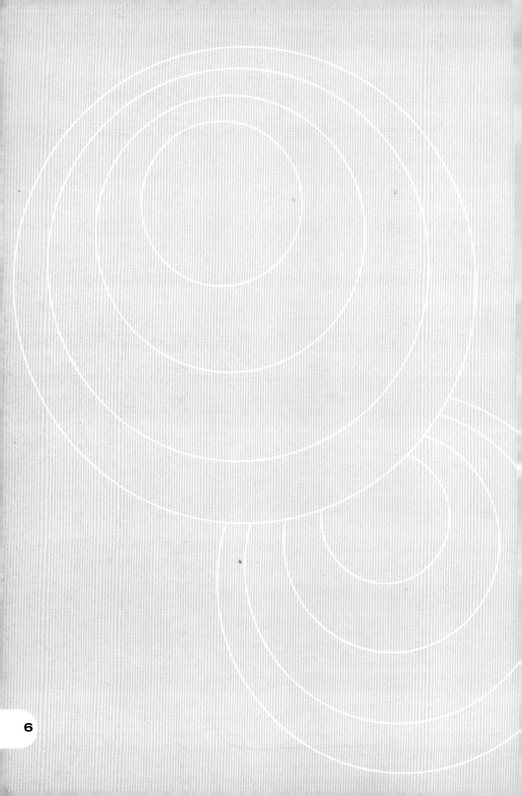

Women are starting to look after themselves at a much earlier age so they can look as good as they can, for as long as they can. They crave information on the latest and greatest miracle creams and wrinkle remedies. Now, for the price of a lipstick, girls can get the real scoop on their biggest beauty concern – wrinkles. This comprehensive guide delivers fresh solutions to the age-old problem of frown and smile lines, furrows, crow's-feet and creases, from the forehead down to the décolleté – for prevention, maintenance and correction. It features the lowdown on the most state-of-the-art methods, what works and what is a waste of money, top clinical advances, new para-surgical treatments, DIY home remedies, as well as resources for how to find a good doctor, shopping guides and web links.

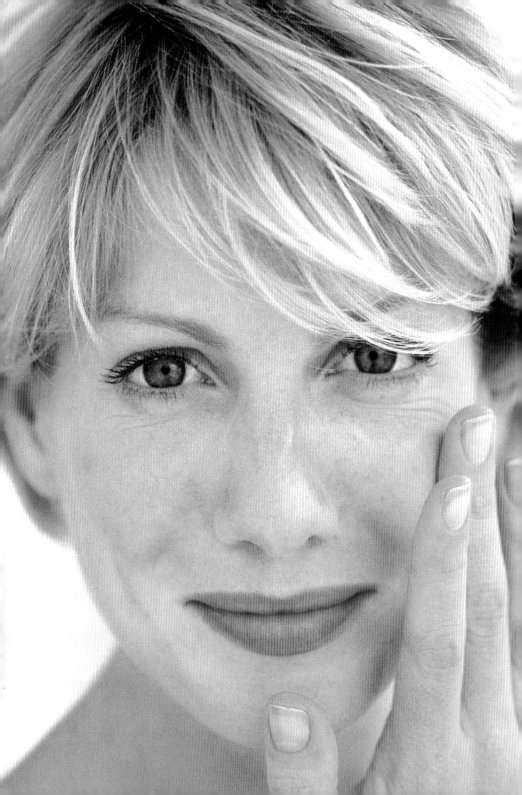

THE BASICS

Our life expectancy has reached an all time high. Women born in 1970 can expect to live an average of 79.5 years. The sad fact is that we all age, but looking older than you have to is a matter of choice. With modern technology, you can hold off looking old for longer.

Wrinkles form largely because levels of collagen — a component of the connective tissue in the skin that creates flexibility — decrease over time. There are two major ways that skin ages: intrinsic ageing, which is genetically programmed and affects the skin all over your body; photoageing, resulting from the long-term effects of sun, smoking and pollution. The degree to which skin photoages is also determined genetically to some extent. Fair-skinned people tend to photoage more and earlier than those with dark skin.

The earlier you start caring for your complexion, the better it will serve you over the long haul. Anti-wrinkle treatments can undo damage, but prevention is best. 80 per cent of the lines and wrinkles you see in the mirror were caused by the sun. The other 20 per cent result from smiling, pouting and frowning. If you have not paid your skin its due respect, all is not lost. It is never too late to start preventing wrinkles, or to begin therapy to soften the ones you have.

face facts

The skin that gets exposed to those nasty UV rays the most – your face, neck and hands – is obviously the part of the body that will age fastest.

Similarly, the skin that is the thinnest on the body – the delicate eyelid area – is most susceptible to damage, lines and ageing. The skin is the body's first defence against disease and infection. It is the largest organ in the body and protects your internal organs from injuries. It regulates body temperature, prevents excess fluid loss and helps your body remove any water and salt that it doesn't need. It also protects against light, infection and environmental elements.

The skin is the body's largest organ, weighing 6–9 pounds and stretching up to 20 square feet. Each square inch of it contains about 15 feet of blood vessels, 10 oil glands and 2 different kinds of sweat glands. The process of producing healthy new skin cells and removing or shedding old cells takes about 28 days.

Thinning skin is a result of a breakdown of collagen fibres. Skin loses elasticity, especially if it has been exposed to excessive sunlight, and becomes more fragile.

Skin deep

Skin is composed of 3 layers: the outermost layer, or epidermis, the middle layer, or dermis, and the deepest layer, the hypodermis.

EPIDERMIS

The epidermis consists of 4 layers: **Stratum corneum** - Dead, dense protein cells known as keratin make up the outer layer of the epidermis that can be seen and felt. **Granular layer** - Dead keratin cells are moved to the surface of the epidermis by the granular layer. **Squamous cell layer** - This layer produces keratin for the stratum corneum and transports water. Blisters originate in the squamous cell layer. **Basal cell layer** - The lowest layer of the epidermis where squamous cells are produced, and the cells that produce melanin, or skin pigment, reside.

DERMIS

The dermis is the middle layer of skin. It is a combination of blood vessels, hair follicles and sebaceous or oil glands. The proteins collagen and elastin are also found in the dermis and provide support and elasticity to the skin. The sun's rays eventually break down these proteins.

HYPODERMIS

The hypodermis is a layer of fatty tissue that provides nourishment to the dermis and upper layers of skin. It also conserves body heat and cushions internal organs against trauma. Blood vessels, nerves, sweat glands and deeper hair follicles are found in the hypodermis.

skin ageing

So you think your skin is going to look young forever. Guess again! At 30, it takes on a life of its own. Your mission is to outsmart your skin cells before they get the better of you.

20s

Skin heaven – Your skin is clear of spots, your pores are invisible and your complexion is even and taut. Save your skin by using an SPF15 everyday and getting your tan out of a bottle, tube or spray. Start your preventative anti-ageing regime with a good eye cream to hold off crow's-feet. Cleanse well, remove all traces of dirt and make-up before going to bed and keep oil plugs at bay with good exfoliation.

30s

Party's over – Expect to see visible changes in your skin's texture. This can be a real eye opener. Cell turnover gently slows down, so adding exfoliants to speed it up is key. It's the perfect time to start more intense anti-ageing skin care. Collagen and elastin fibres begin to break down, so keep them firm by integrating nutrients into your programme like Vitamin C, AHAs, antioxidants and plant enzymes. Smokers will start to see fine lines around the mouth and squinters will spy their first crow's-feet. It's the ideal time to get professional advice about treatments like BOTOX®, peeling treatments and lasers for thread veins.

40s

They're here – Your wrinkles are in full force so it's time to bring out the heavy artillery. Everything becomes lazy: skin gets drier, sagging and wrinkles give way to folds, furrows and creases. Your brow droops and the corners of your mouth turn down as jowls creep up. The best plan is to fight back with medically advanced skin care formulas which are worth spending money on. Look for high-tech ingredients like antioxidants and enzymes, which should keep your face and neck supple. Wage war on brown spots with lightening agents. Stick to a regime of facial peels, BOTOX® and wrinkle fillers to combat creases. This is the time to start investigating surgical options to plan for your beauty future.

50s

Desperate measures – It's a big number, but don't let it get you down. Turn back the clock with rejuvenating treatments, moisturizing serums and firming masks. Your hormones are wreaking havoc, accounting for enlarged pores and increased oil activity. At this stage, you will get limited results from para-surgical treatments. Once your jawline starts to soften and the nasal labial folds require lots of filling, the time has come to nip or tuck. Facelift techniques have come a long way. With shorter scars and faster healing, they are the mainstay in a woman's arsenal against ageing. By having your first lift before you turn 50 you may never have to go public. It won't make you look 25 again but it can keep your big birthday a secret for longer.

all dried up

Facial skin typically looks its best during a woman's 20s. As you age, your skin becomes thinner and often drier. It will also make less natural oil, which can make wrinkling more apparent.

Skin dries out because the structure weakens and it doesn't retain moisture as well as younger skin. With the menopause come declining oestrogen levels. Skin usually gets drier, however some women become oilier even if they never had oily skin as a teenager. The skin may also be affected by diuretics and certain medications such as those for blood pressure.

Dry skin may suggest that your skin is lacking the nutrients it needs to stay healthy. Topical agents such as wrinkle creams and moisturizers help give the top layer of skin the Vitamins and minerals that can help this layer look younger and healthier. Not every face needs a moisturizer and of those that do, not all require daily applications. If your skin is dry, moisturize it. The drier it is, the heavier the moisturizer you need. If your skin is naturally oily, there is no need to add extra moisture to it. The amount of natural lubrication or sebum produced by the skin declines with age.

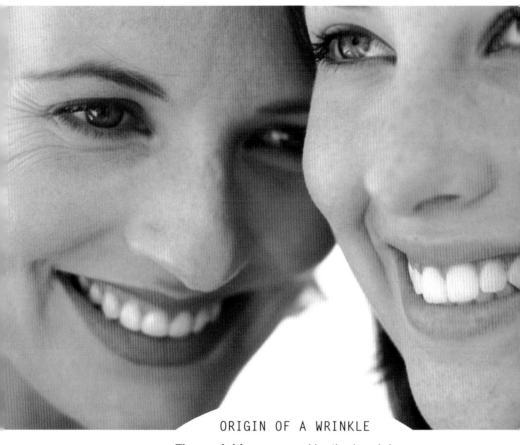

ORIGIN OF A WRINKLE

Fine wrinkles - caused by the breakdown
of collagen and elastin fibres over time.

Deep wrinkles - caused by the building up of muscle in
the deeper layers below the surface of the skin.

Dynamic wrinkles - only visible when muscles are
engaged, as in smiling or frowning.

Static wrinkles - seen all the time, when
the face is at rest or moving.

maintenance

Preserving a healthy, youthful appearance involves maintenance, a lifestyle approach to prolonging youthful, gorgeous skin for as long as possible through sensible living, advanced skin care, occasional beauty shots and skin treatments.

The factors that may determine how long your skin will stay glowing include genetics, your diet and nutrition, sun exposure, whether you smoke or drink heavily and your stress levels. The best defence you've got is to protect your skin from free radical damage and make use of therapies that go on a search and destroy mission to neutralize the little molecules.

Hot water and soap dissolve the skin's natural moisture, so if your skin is dry, keep your daily shower short and water temperature moderate. While bathing, rub your body with a flannel to exfoliate the skin. Gently pat yourself dry. If you rub too hard at either point, you may remove too much skin and contribute to further dehydration. While the skin is still damp, apply a moisturizer. Moisturizers don't usually last all day, so reapplication may be necessary. In general, the heavier the moisturizer, the better it works on dry skin. When the skin becomes dry it needs water to help rejuvenate it, and moisturizers act to trap water in the skin. Relief for dry skin typically comes in these forms: ointments, creams, oils and lotions.

Ointments

Thick, greasy and best for preventing moisture from escaping from the skin. These are inconvenient for regular use. Ointments are best saved for areas that take a lot of abuse such as hands, elbows and feet.

Creams

Heavier than lotions and more effective at sealing in moisture for normal to dry skin.

Oils

Easily absorbed when applied to slightly damp skin after you pat dry, but often less moisturizing than ointments, creams or lotions.

Lotions

Thinner and lighter so least effective at replacing lost moisture in very dry skin. They evaporate quickly, making them the most convenient to use. They are often preferred over ointments and creams because they apply and absorb more easily. They are good for normal, oily and younger skin types that don't need as much added hydration. Lotions are also generally good for the body, but are less effective at sealing moisture in than ointments or creams.

TOP TIP:

A quick fix approach to skin care is destined to fail. Take the time to get educated and don't be afraid to ask for help when you need it.

clean regime

Skin problems can be prevented or minimized by following a good skin care programme that has been specifically designed for your skin type, condition and concern.

Repairing skin that has visible signs of ageing will not happen overnight. It is like starting an exercise programme – start slow, gradually increasing your tolerance in stages. As with exercise, if you stop, the problem comes back again. Every woman is constantly looking for the perfect skin care regime; a cleanser that removes make-up and leaves your skin feeling comfortable, a toner that refreshes without drying you out and a moisturizer that keeps you hydrated without clogging pores. There is no such thing. A great skin care regime involves more than one product and varies from one face to another. Eye creams are specially formulated for delicate eyelid skin. Some face and neck formulas will be too heavy around the eyes. If your eyes are puffy, use a lighter formula. Thicker ones will trap too much moisture in the skin and cause swelling.

Minimum maintenance
by day:
Cleanser
Eye cream
Moisturizer with SPF15

Minimum maintenance
by night:
Cleanser
Toner (optional)
Eye cream
Night cream

five easy steps

1 **Cleanse (and tone)** – Any dermatologist will tell you to use a basic, gentle non-detergent cleanser and make sure to rinse off all residue. You only need to use a toner if your skin doesn't feel clean without it, you are in a humid atmosphere or you have oily or acne prone skin.

2 **Exfoliate** – All skins need some form of exfoliation, but the degree will differ.

3 **Treat** – This phase encompasses everything from treating acne, eczema, bleaching dark spots, to oil control and anti-ageing.

4 **Moisturize** – Skin needs hydration, but not all skin needs the same amount. Oily skin needs less and may not need any in particularly spot prone areas. The eyelid area needs the most because it has the fewest oil glands.

5 **Protect** – Every skin needs sun protection daily, all year long. When trying a new skin care product, you should use it regularly for at least a month before evaluating its effectiveness. Your skin fluctuates with your monthly menstrual cycle. In order to determine whether a product works for you, you'll need to use it during each phase of that cycle. Don't try more than one new product at a time, as it will be hard to tell how your skin responds to any of them.

changing times

Keeping on top of your skin care regime means altering it as your skin changes, with the seasons, and depending on the climate you live in.

In autumn and winter, exposure to cold weather outside and hot, dry air inside can cause skin to lose moisture rapidly. In the spring and summer months, extra heat and moisture in the air can lead to oilier skin and increased perspiration, even in people who normally have dry skin. Most women make the mistake of over-moisturizing, when and where it isn't needed. Overloading the skin can clog pores and keep dead cells from sloughing off.

It's time to change your skin care routine

- When you're under stress
- When you're going on holiday
- When the climate changes
- Seasonally
- With every decade
- As your skin shows visible changes

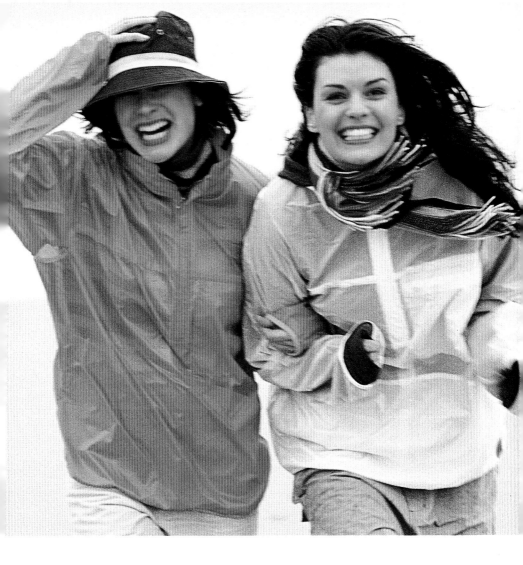

Timed to perfection

For normal skin, facial treatments can be scheduled for every 8 weeks. If your skin is environmentally challenged, bump that up to every 4-6 weeks. For oily skin in need of deep cleansing, every 3-4 weeks might be better. If you have acne, don't overdo it. Let your skin be the judge.

PREVENTING THEM

An ounce of prevention is worth many pounds in future wrinkle remedies. The best way to deal with wrinkles is not to get them in the first place. Protecting the skin from the sun is the single most important practice in skin care. Continuous exposure to the sun's rays will wrinkle and dry out the skin, leaving it coarse and thick. Uneven pigmentation, freckles for example, is another side effect of sunning. The earliest warning sign of severe skin damage is the development of 'actinic keratoses'. These pre-cancerous lesions affect approximately 1 in 6 people. They are most common in people with fair skin and light hair, but can affect anybody who has been overly exposed to the sun.

As you get older, your cumulative sun damage will start to crop up on you even if you thought you had outsmarted it. The sun's rays are very unforgiving and the damage they do to the skin is inescapable. Products used for prevention don't necessarily produce visible results. For example, your sunscreen won't reduce wrinkles, but consistent use will stop them from forming as quickly and as deeply.

the inside out

Foods high in vitamins C and E (like onions, garlic, fish, peas, beans, dark green leafy vegetables and whole grains), won't keep you wrinkle-free, but evidence suggests they can help.

- **Water** – drink 6–8 glasses per day to keep skin hydrated.

- **Fruits and vegetables** – a diet rich in these will naturally be high in antioxidants.

- **Complex carbohydrates** – found in whole grains, oatmeal and fruits, they should supply 50 per cent of your calories.

- **Lean protein** – your skin needs approximately 44 g per day to produce collagen.

- **Recommended Daily Amounts (RDA)** – these vary from person to person, so consult your doctor or nutritionist. Smokers and drinkers may need more. If you are deficient in any nutrients, take a supplement as well as following a healthy diet.

- **Maximum RDAs for women** – vit. A: 1.5 mg, vit. C: 1200 mg, vit. E: 20 mg, Selenium: 55 mcg, Calcium: 1500 mg, Thiamine: 1.5 mg, Zinc: 15 mg, Linoleic acid: 2 g, Alpha Linolenic acid: 0.5 g.

- **Caffeine and alcohol** – avoid these, or keep them to a minimum.

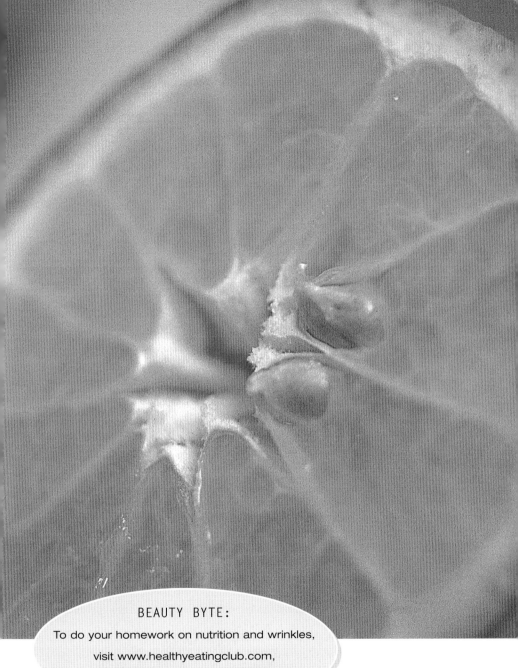

BEAUTY BYTE:

To do your homework on nutrition and wrinkles,

visit www.healthyeatingclub.com,

www.realage.com and www.thirdage.com

free radicals

When it comes to your complexion, free radicals are one of the things that make the difference between peaches 'n' cream and wrinkled prune.

Free radicals are the by-products formed when oxygen is used by the body. They weave their damage by annihilating collagen and elastin fibres, cell membranes and DNA. Antioxidants protect precious pores by going on a search and destroy mission to neutralize free radicals. They assist in skin repair and the strengthening of blood vessels. It's a clear battle of good versus evil.

Free radicals start a chain reaction under the skin's surface. The skin is damaged and its cellular structure is weakened. They alter the DNA, resulting in ageing and illness. Stress produces adrenaline-related products, which restrict blood flow to the skin and generate free radicals. Ageing is caused by the slow cumulative oxidation of body tissues over a lifetime. Free radicals affect the rate at which we age generally, plus research has pointed the finger at them as the cause of some cancers, heart disease, arthritis, Alzheimer's and Parkinson's Disease.

The body makes its own antioxidants to deal with free radicals, but an overload caused by sun or smoking could leave the body unable to cope. Skin thickness increases with age, while skin elasticity decreases. Unfortunately, this cannot be avoided. Ensuring that your antioxidant levels remain high is healthy, but they can't correct the loss of elasticity, eliminate wrinkles or make skin look significantly younger. At present, research is inconclusive.

Antioxidants

The best way to get your antioxidants is from food first, supplements last.

TOP TIP:

Ingestion of large amounts of some vitamins can be toxic. Don't overdo it. Follow the Upper Level guidelines for every supplement you take.

Carotenoids

The basic function of carotenoids is as a source of vitamin A.

Alpha and beta-carotene – found in orange and yellow fruits and vegetables such as carrots, pumpkin, yellow squash, apricots and mangoes and in dark green leafy vegetables like spinach and parsley.

Lycopene – the red pigment in tomatoes, watermelon and pink grapefruit.

Lutein and Zeaxanthin – found in green leafy vegetables like spinach and yellow and orange fruits and vegetables such as squash.

Beta – Cryptoxanthin – found in mangoes, red capsicum and pumpkin.

Flavonoids

Found in tea – especially green tea – onions, red wine and red grape juice.

Vitamin C

Found in fruit and vegetables, including oranges, blackcurrants, strawberries, grapefruit, kiwi fruit, potatoes and peas.

Vitamin E

Found in the fatty parts of foods, safflower oil, margarine, mayonnaise, wheat germ, nuts and seeds, with smaller amounts in most fruit and vegetables.

ray bans

Approximately 5 per cent of the UV radiation hitting the skin is reflected. The remaining 95 per cent passes into the tissue, gets scattered and then passes out again, or gets absorbed by molecules in the various layers of the epidermis and dermis.

UVA rays are longer than UVB so they can penetrate more deeply through the skin's surface where they kill collagen and elastin, which makes your skin slack and floppy, and cause dry, leathery, blotchy skin. How wrinkled your skin gets depends largely on how much sun you have been exposed to in your lifetime. People who spend a lot of time outside without adequate protection, develop leathery skin earlier, which makes them look older than they are.

Light spectrum

The longer the wavelength the greater the energy level and the more damage it can do.

UVA – Longer wavelengths mostly transmitted to the dermis to be absorbed by haemoglobin in the blood or reflected back up and out of the body; known to cause damage in the deeper layers, and skin cancer.

UVB – Shorter wavelengths largely removed in the epidermis, particularly by DNA and melanin; known to cause sunburn and skin cancer.

UV radiation has many effects on the skin as a result of its absorption by skin molecules, called chromophores, the most important of which is DNA. After UV absorption, DNA undergoes chemical changes. If these alterations are not repaired, they can be highly disruptive to the way cells function. It is now known that even small amounts of sunlight on the skin can cause DNA damage throughout the entire thickness of the epidermis. Fortunately, most of this is repaired within days, although some permanent damage may remain. The absorption of UV radiation by skin chromophores and the unrepaired damage are considered the main causes of visible skin damage. All levels of the skin are affected, but because UVB is largely absorbed high up before it reaches the dermis, most of the immediate damage is to the epidermis. UVA makes up approximately 95 per cent of the ultraviolet light that we are exposed to.

When DNA is damaged by UVB exposure, chemicals are released that are important in repairing other skin molecular structures and which cause underlying blood vessels to swell. This is what shows up as sunburn. These chemicals may also contribute to harming the collagen and elastin fibres in the dermis, helping to speed up ageing. If after severe sunburn, the damage is so extensive that the cell cannot repair itself and dies, the skin blisters and peels. If the DNA is not accurately repaired, it is possible that the cells may pass on a mutation that may eventually lead to skin cancer.

REALITY CHECK:
Longer UVA and UVB wavelengths can pass right through the atmosphere even on a cloudy day, so you can still get sunburnt when the sun isn't shining.

photoageing

To judge the effects of photoageing on your skin, compare the appearance of areas that have not been exposed to the sun, with your face, hands and chest.

Those areas normally covered by clothing are smoother and tend to be more freckle and wrinkle free. Facial skin, in contrast, may be freckled or dry and often looks dull, blotchy and deeply wrinkled. It can also become covered with thread veins.

Photoageing is the result of accumulated skin damage caused by UV radiation over many years. As with sunburn, UVB wavelengths have the greatest impact. The potentially deeper reaching UVA rays may affect you if you spend a lot of time on a sunbed or sunbathing, using a sunscreen that only blocks UVB rays. When the body is unable to fully repair damage to the DNA in the cells of the epidermis and the dermis, their structure deteriorates. The changes can be irreversible. Sunlight also causes changes to the melanocytes, which gradually stop functioning so that your skin develops brown spots, blotchiness or a yellowish hue. The epidermis becomes thinner and more fragile. All these changes together make up the visible signs of skin photoageing.

REALITY CHECK:
The only safe tan is a fake tan. Tanning parlours are public enemy number one and a wrinkle's best friend.

Never too early to start

Start your sun protection programme early: it has been estimated that up to 50 per cent of your total UV radiation exposure is acquired by the age of 18, and 75 per cent by the age of 30.

If your photoageing clock has been ticking for some time, you can minimize further changes by being careful in the sun from now on. Photoageing steadily develops even if you avoid sunbathing. Simply taking a walk around the block or sitting at a street café will allow your skin to be affected by the sun's rays. The skin doesn't need to turn red, pink or burn for slow permanent damage to take place. Sunburn is a skin repair process. Tanning is the release of UV-protective pigment following UV-induced DNA damage. Accumulated skin damage over many years produces deep wrinkles. Although the skin on your face may never look as young as the skin on your buttocks, it will look much better if you protect it from sun exposure. Practicing safe sun and avoiding tanning beds are a MUST.

SEVEN SIGNS OF PHOTOAGEING

- Dehydrated and thickened outer skin layers
- Flaking and rough skin
- Age spots and sunburn freckles
- Sallow complexion
- Enlarged pores clogged with sebum
- Broken, enlarged capillaries
- Milia or small white cysts

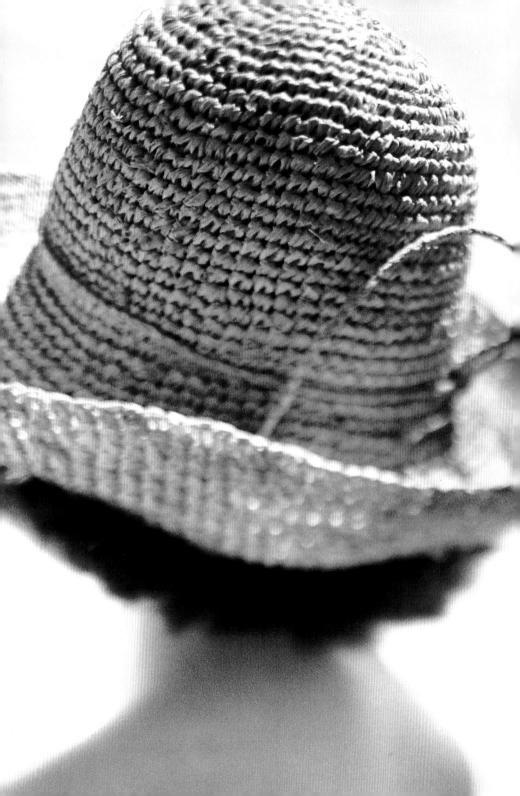

spf savvy

Sunscreens temporarily absorb ultraviolet rays. The best formulas protect against both UVA – the culprit in wrinkle formation – and UVB, which causes tanning and burning.

The higher the Sun Protection Factor (SPF) rating, the stronger and longer its effects. The SPF index only addresses UVB rays. For protection against UVA, look for products containing Parsol 1789, zinc oxide, or titanium dioxide.

TOP TIP: When it comes to suntan lotion, rub it on, rub it in well, rub it all over and rub it often.

The burning question is 'how much do I really need?' Sunblock should come in a 6-pack, because most of us use far too little of it to be effective. Very few people use sunscreen everyday, all year round. Autumn and winter are no exception, no matter where you live or travel to.

Screen versus block

Sunscreen - chemical agent that denatures light, making the wavelengths incapable of causing damage.

Sunblock - agent that acts as a physical barrier to prevent sunlight from reaching the surface of the skin.

Some sunscreen formulas combine a mixture of the two concepts. More sensitive skin types may tolerate physical blockers better. Sunscreens with a heavier coating provide a better physical barrier.

screening room

Does your sun protection pass the test? With so many formulas on the market, it's hard to know which one is best for you.

Always use a minimum of SPF15. Use SPF30 for more intense exposure. Choose products that offer broad spectrum protection (both UVA and UVB). For spot-prone skin, use an oil-free or non-comedogenic sunscreen.

There are two types of sunscreens:
Chemicals - absorb UV light to reduce the amount that reaches the skin.

Reflectors - derived from minerals like titanium dioxide and zinc oxide that scatter sunlight thus reflecting it away from the skin.

Sunscreens with physical blockers, which lie on the skin's surface, are widely available. The new mineral sunscreens are lighter and wearable under make-up. Zinc oxide is the more potent and more expensive, so titanium dioxide is more widely used.

The difference in texture between cosmetic sunscreens for daily protection and sport sunscreens for outdoor and beach protection is waterproofing. Waterproof lotions have an oil base, which is thicker and heavier and can clog pores. When a product is labelled 'water resistant', it should specify the length of time it will last if you come into contact

TOP TIP:

The best sun protectors are a
wide-brimmed hat and protective
clothing, especially the kind made
with cool, light, tightly woven fabrics
that keep the sun's rays out.
Sunglasses with polarized lenses
offer protection for your eyes
and from crow's-feet.

with water. Labelling varies from country to country and there is still no standardization. Many derma-tologists believe that over SPF15, the differences in protection levels are very small, but SPF15 is the minimum you need for it to be effective. Bump that up to SPF30 if you are playing sports, or are on a holiday where you are outdoors more than usual, skiing, swimming or strolling.

Using a moisturizer that contains a sunscreen can also be misleading. You are unlikely to apply as much of it or use it as often as a regular sunscreen, so it will not be as effective. It may be adequate if you apply it all over your face and neck daily, if your sun exposure is limited. It would not be considered enough protection for a day at the beach or playing tennis. What you use on your body is not the same as what you would choose for your face. Most women tend to buy two different sun products; one for the body and one with a higher SPF for the face. Choose a moderately priced formula for your body so you'll use more of it. It is critical that you like the feel, fragrance and texture, to ensure that you use it daily. For your face, splurge on an elegant product that you enjoy using.

TOP TIP:

Don't forget to cover
the most burn-prone
areas: your lips, eyelids,
back of neck, tip of nose,
forehead, chest,
shoulders and ears.

the best protection

The ideal sunscreen for you is one that will provide the necessary level of protection for your skin type, degree of sun exposure and risk for sun sensitivity.

A fair blonde who is going on holiday to the Caribbean generally needs more protection than an olive skinned brunette walking down the high street in March. The key is that whatever your sunscreen of choice, you must use enough of it and use it regularly. Dermatologists recommend using 30 g or 1 oz of lotion for one person's whole body, per application.

Great foundations

Even if a foundation contains a sunscreen, facial movements throughout the day remove some of it from your face, decreasing its effectiveness. Foundations, concealers, moisturizers, eye creams and lipsticks that offer UVA and UVB protection may be sufficient for normal daily activities. Sebum is produced during the day, thus separating the foundation from the skin's surface. Everyone experiences this, but normal to dry skin types will find it develops at a slower rate. When you are outside for a long period, your foundation will only protect you for about 2 hours. After that, either reapply foundation or use a sunscreen over it for continued protection.

TOP TIP:
If you are using a separate sunscreen for the face, apply it evenly all over the face and neck, under make-up.

Suncare lingo

SPF (Sun Protection Factor) – the ratio of the amount of energy from the sun's rays that it takes to turn sunscreen-protected skin red, compared with the energy it takes if the skin is unprotected.

PABA (Para Aminobenzoic Acid) – a UVB-absorbing ingredient that was commonly used in sunscreens in the past. Becase it can cause irritation and reactions, it is not used for the most part today. PABA-free formulas are easier to tolerate.

Chemical sunscreens – UV absorbers
Avobenzone (Parsol 1789) – provides broad spectrum protection against UVA and UVB rays. Newer formulas combine Parsol 1789 with stabilizing agents to improve its stability in sunlight. Other ingredients include Benzophenone, Dioxybenzone, Menthyl Anthranitate, Octyl Methoxycinnamate and Oxybenzone.

Physical sunscreens – sunblocking agents
Titanium Dioxide and Zinc Oxide are the gold standard. Others include Iron Oxide, Kaolin, Bentonite, Magnesium Silicate, Mica and Talc.

Dihydroxyacetone (DHA) – active ingredient in artificial tanning products that interacts with the proteins in the skin to darken skin temporarily. This is not a sunscreen.

smoke out

You can ALWAYS tell a smoker by her skin. It has a grey or sallow cast, feels dry, and is usually lined prematurely – early to mid 30s – especially around the mouth and eyes.

Even if you only have a few cigarettes a day, expect the telltale wrinkles around the mouth and eyes to appear in your 30s. Scientists have an explanation for what makes smokers look old before their time. Tobacco has been found to activate the genes responsible for the skin enzyme that breaks down collagen, the protein that maintains elasticity in the skin. When this starts to disintegrate, the skin begins to sag and wrinkle. Too much of the enzyme increases the ageing effect of the sun's ultraviolet rays, which also raises the concentration of the enzyme. Smokers are more prone to getting wrinkles and their skin tends to have a greyish pallor. Smoking causes a flood of free radicals to form in the body, which speeds up the ageing process. Research suggests that smokers have lower levels of vitamin C in their blood than nonsmokers, and that their daily loss of vitamin C is about 35 mg/day greater than nonsmokers. Women who smoke need to consume at least 110 mg/day of Vitamin C to compensate for this loss.

The combination of smoking and sunlight is positively deadly. Plus the nicotine stains on your teeth and fingers are far from glamorous. The best beauty treatment and the cheapest by far is to QUIT SMOKING.

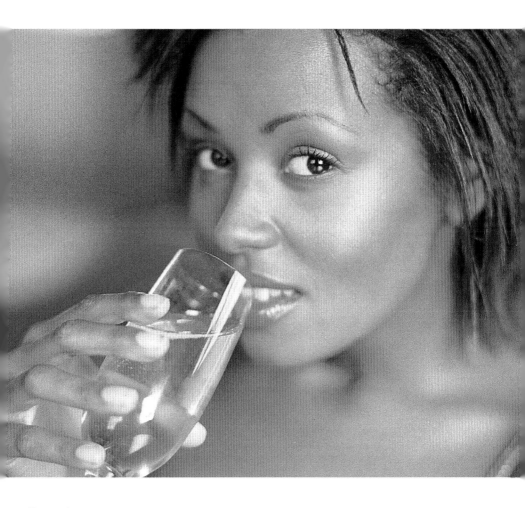

Drunken pores

Want great skin? Then steer clear of over-indulging on skin-aggravating alcohol. Aside from hangovers, alcohol can wreak havoc on your skin. High alcohol consumption can cause a puffy face, red and irritated eyes and a washed out complexion. Alcohol is a diuretic and causes blood vessels to dilate and the skin to lose moisture, resulting in dehydration, sagging and a loss of resiliency. To help skin stay wrinkle free, keep cocktails to a minimum.

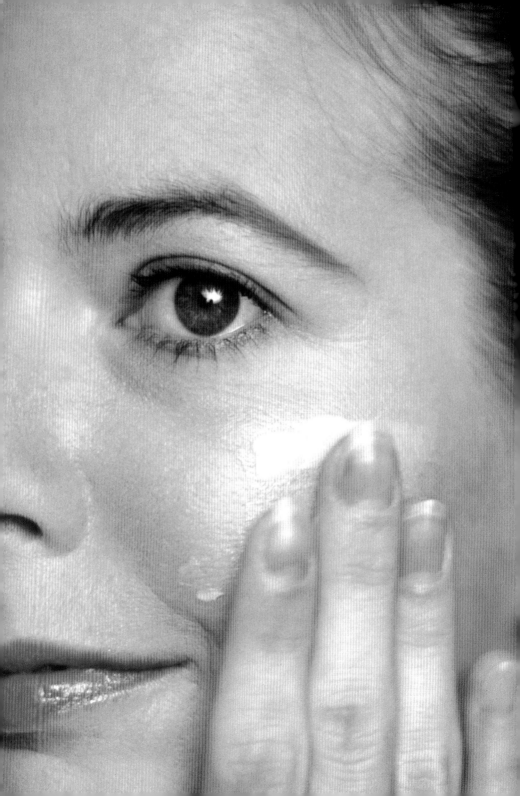

SMOOTHING THEM

SMOOTHING THEM

The ageing process is under intense scrutiny by the scientific community. Every skin care product today has some combination of vitamins. The trick is to look for high concentrations of vitamins like B, E, C and K and other antioxidants, and to ensure that they are used in stable enough forms to be applied topically. Retinoic acid, L-ascorbic acid and alpha hydroxy acids have been thought of as the mainstays for aeons, but that's just the start. While they tackle skin ageing in scientifically different ways, they work synergistically when used together. L-ascorbic acid is often recommended for daytime use as it acts as a sunscreen safety net. The trend is to develop increasingly potent skin care treatments with higher levels of active ingredients, but with fewer of the side effects associated with high tech formulations.

Exfoliation means to strip away the old to bring in the new. On the skin this translates as radiance, vitality and clarity. As cells clump together, you need to jumpstart the natural process of sloughing off. There are many modern tools for exfoliation, from sponges, loofahs, flannels and wipes, to peeling agents that penetrate the skin.

boosters

If you're approaching 30, consider adding a few 'active' products to your skin care programme to make sure you reap the benefits of today's advanced technologies.

The term 'active' describes a product containing an ingredient that works beneath the skin's surface, producing visible changes. The active substance should appear in the first 3–5 ingredients on the list. For an ingredient to work it has to: be protected from air and light, reach the target tissue in an active form, be delivered in a high enough concentration to be effective and be used on a regular basis.

Anti-ageing skin care formulations fall into three classifications: over-the-counter (cosmetics); non-prescription (cosmeceuticals); prescription (drugs). Cosmeceuticals includes bioactives that have anti-ageing, moisturizing, firming and skin lightening effects. The cosmeceutical category is considered the most scientifically reliable and potent because the products generally contain the highest concentrations of active ingredients.

Beauty and the lab

The key in this age of product overload is to read labels. New compounds are turning up in cleansers, moisturizers and sunscreens all the time. It's hard to keep up, especially when some ingredients go by more than one name. By law, the first ingredient listed on the label should have the highest concentration in the formula, but every ingredient is listed, even when there are only trace amounts of it in the product.

Skin vitamins

Arnica - A botanical derived from a mountain plant, with antiseptic, astringent, antimicrobial and anti-inflammatory properties.

Copper peptides - Known to aid in the healing of wounds.

Gluconolactone - One of the poly hydroxy acids that occurs naturally jn the cells.

Hyaluronic acid - A polysaccharide naturally found in the body's connective tissues, used as a moisturizing agent in cosmetics.

Lactobionic acid - Contains gluconic acid, one of the poly hydroxy acids, found to aid in wound-healing and decreasing scaling.

L-ascorbic acid - Also referred to as vitamin C, a water-soluble antioxidant, known for its ability to destroy free radicals.

L-Glutathione - Found in all human tissues, a potent antioxidant amino acid that accelerates wound healing.

Linoleic acid - A liquid essential fatty acid that acts as a moisturizing agent.

Panthenol - Vitamin B5, a humectant that attracts water to the dermis to increase hydration.

Retinyl palmitate - A vitamin A derived essential skin nutrient for healthy skin maintenance and repair.

Tea tree oil - A natural preservative with antiseptic and germicidal properties, also used in acne preparations.

Vitamin K - Used to lessen redness and reduce the appearance of broken capillaries and bruising.

acid test

AHAs are a group of acids from fruit and other natural substances, that speed cell turnover and improve texture, reduce fine lines and even out skin tone.

AHAs are key to unclogging embedded cellular debris from pores and shedding the outermost layer of dead skin. They work by consistently peeling away dead and thickened areas of the skin, in essence thinning the build-up. If you stop using AHAs, your skin's turnover rate will gradually become more sluggish. With continued use, AHAs have been proven to improve a wide range of skin conditions including wrinkles, acne, blotches and age spots.

In 1997, the Cosmetic Ingredient Review Panel concluded that AHAs and their related compounds are safe, when the concentration is 10 per cent or less, the final product has a pH of 3.5 or greater and the product is formulated to protect the skin from increased sun sensitivity or is used with a sunscreen. Over-the-counter AHA strengths vary from 4 to 15 per cent, but are often neutralized to a degree that they are not very effective – 8 per cent is considered the baseline level needed to see results. You will only see visible improvement for as long as you are using the product. The more buffered the formula, the gentler it is. AHAs have the potential for irritation if you use the wrong strength or too much of the right one. Most skin types can

WARNING: If you have rosacea or very sensitive skin, AHAs may increase redness and cause stinging, irritation and flare-ups.

Natural exfoliants

Glycolic acid – Most common AHA, derived from sugar cane and can also be made from synthetic ingredients. Because it is a small molecule, it penetrates the skin easily.

Malic acid – Derived from apples and white grapes.

Tartaric acid - A type of glycolic acid that results from the fermentation process used in making wine.
Uses: exfoliation; reducing surface oils; unclogging blackheads; smoothing fine lines

Beta hydroxy acid – Primarily used to exfoliate the epidermis and prevent clogged pores. It is also referred to as salicylic acid. It does not penetrate as deeply into the dermis as glycolic acid, so it is less irritating.

Citric acid – Derived from citrus fruits. Acts as an antioxidant on the skin.
Uses: may stimulate collagen production; has mild bleaching properties

Lactic acid – Comes from sour milk. Works as an exfoliator and to hold water in the skin as a component of the skin's natural moisturizing mechanism.
Uses: softening thick, rough skin; moisturizing

Polyhydroxy acids – Considered one of the mildest formulations because they are larger molecules so are limited in the way they can penetrate the skin.
Uses: softening thick, rough skin; moisturizing

use some form, but very sensitive skin types may only be able to tolerate the mildest like polyhydroxy acids.

As the skin becomes conditioned to hydroxy acids, stronger concentrations can be used for a deeper exfoliation. Follow your programme daily, or twice a day if your skin can tolerate it, to avoid the build-up of keratin and dead cells, and to help moisturizers to penetrate more deeply.

sloughing off

When you hit 30 and your skin can't slough off its outer layer as easily and uniformly as it once did, it can begin to look dull. Products are available to give your skin some assistance.

Tretinoin

Scientific data on retinoic acid for treating and preventing photoageing, has inspired a generation of newcomers that offer similar properties with less flaking, redness and irritation. Retinoic acid acts as a chemical peeling agent that helps the skin to renew itself more rapidly. It does have the potential to irritate so if you have a reaction to it, try skipping a day, using it every 2 days or just applying it to wrinkle prone areas like crow's-feet, forehead lines and around the lips. You can also experiment with 'short contact therapy', i.e. using a thin coat and washing it off after 10 minutes, so the drug penetration is limited. The key is to start with a low concentration and work your way up until you reach the highest concentration that your skin can tolerate. Then use this on a regular basis. Tretinoin is used in concentrations of 0.025, 0.05 and 0.01 per cent and microencapsulated forms.

Tretinoin emollient cream

This prescription cream is basically Retin-A® in a moisturizing base that decreases the redness and burning. Renova® or Retinova® is prescription strength Retin-A® in a mineral oil base that is ideally suited to dry, ageing skin. It has the distinction of being the only product approved by the US Food and Drug Administration for the treatment of wrinkles. It should be applied exactly as your doctor prescribes, usually once a day at bedtime. Do not apply more cream or use it more often than stated by your doctor. Your wrinkles will not go away any faster and the skin may become severely irritated. Renova® may be too rich or creamy for you if your skin is oily or acne-prone. Tretinoin emollient cream is available in concentrations of 0.02 and 0.05 per cent.

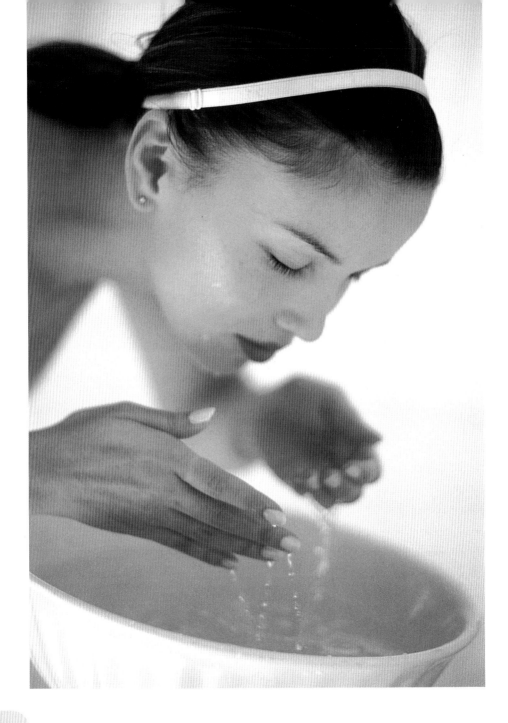

retinols

The next step is retinol (called trans-retinol), which is an over-the-counter vitamin A derivative that stimulates cell division and can reduce fine lines over time.

Research suggests that small amounts of retinol can function as an antioxidant. It gets converted by the skin to retinoic acid, the main ingredient in Retin-A®. The advantage is that it can produce changes in the skin similar to retinoic acid without measurable irritation. Although you won't see results as quickly, a smaller amount of Vitamin A is better than none. Typical over-the-counter formulas contain as little as 0.1 per cent, up to a maximum of 5 per cent.

Good medicine

Instructions for use:

- Before applying the cream, wash your face with mild soap.
- Pat it dry and wait 20–30 minutes before applying the cream.
- Use a pea-sized amount to cover the face.
- Wash your hands after applying it.
- Daily use of an SPF15 is essential.

Possible side effects:

flaking, dryness, stinging, burning, redness, irritation

the A team

Vitamin A, most commonly found in yellow and orange vegetables, has held its place as the leader in the realm of anti-ageing skin care.

Retinoic acid, a pure form of Vitamin A, can reduce fine lines, fade age spots, clear pimples and control rosacea. Originally prescribed for acne, Retin-A® (whose active ingredient is tretinoin) has been found to do much more. It exfoliates the surface of the skin unblocking clogged pores, and forces the cells below to regenerate more quickly. The result is smoother skin thanks to the increase of collagen and elastin fibres. To see visible improvement, you have to use it for at least a month and the improvement will last only as long as it is used. It also makes the skin more sun-sensitive, so sun protection and avoiding sunlamps is vital. Side effects include redness, dryness and sensitivity.

TOP TIP:
If you're a first time user, don't buy cosmeceuticals online unless you have been advised by a skin care professional. If you are a novice, always start with the mildest formula and work your way up.

WARNING: You should not use retinoid creams on sunburn, eczema or other skin conditions.

firming them

Some women are religious in their belief that facial exercises and muscle-toning techniques will forestall a face-lift forever. The truth is that nothing can eliminate the need for a face-lift.

At some point, the ageing process catches up with all of us, and when jowls start sagging, the scalpel is the only way to go. Facial exercises may not be all that beneficial to sagging skin, nor will they remove your wrinkles. Facial muscles are the only muscles in the body that insert into skin rather than bone. For this reason, 'exercising' them might even worsen wrinkling, especially lines of expression like the creases from the nose to the mouth and forehead folds.

Muscle-toning treatments are touted as the knife-free alternative to a face- or neck-lift. 'Non-surgical face-lift' procedures promise a lot, but usually deliver little. The machines typically use microcurrent therapy to lift and tone the face. Having a treatment before a party may give you a temporary lifting effect, but it will be long since gone by the morning after. Some women continue having maintenance treatments for years. It's called blind faith. Muscle toning is also said to be a preventative procedure, so it is recommended that candidates start in their 30s before the face begins to sag. However, the muscles of the face are the most exercised muscles in the body and additional exercise may only deepen your creases and folds. Don't expect miracles, and don't expect to avoid a face-lift. The only thing that has a significant effect on sagging facial muscles is tightening them via surgery.

antioxidants

Scientists agree that some antioxidants fight off wrinkles from the inside and the outside, but exactly how much you need for them to work is up for debate.

Antioxidants applied to the skin have been studied for their ability to stimulate fibroblast activity, maintain and repair the dermis and help to prevent sun damage. Combining several concentrated forms makes them work harder than they can on their own. Vitamins C and E work wonders as a team. C regenerates E after it has neutralized those pesky free radicals. The new kids on the block are Silymarin (better known as extract of milk thistle), Soya Isoflavones and Green Tea Polyphenols, all powerful antioxidants that protect against UVA and UVB. Green Tea can soothe sunburn, and is 20 times more powerful as an antioxidant than Vitamin C.

Key antioxidants in skin care

Alpha Lipoic Acid – An antioxidant that fights free radicals in the fat and aqueous phases of cells.

Coenzyme Q10 – Ubiquinone, a fat-soluble antioxidant that is close to Vitamin E in structure.

Grape seed oil – An antioxidant with a high linoleic acid content.

Green tea – The polyphenols from green tea can protect skin from UVB damage.

Milk thistle – Also known as silymarin extract, this is a bioflavonoid used for its antioxidant and anti-inflammatory properties.

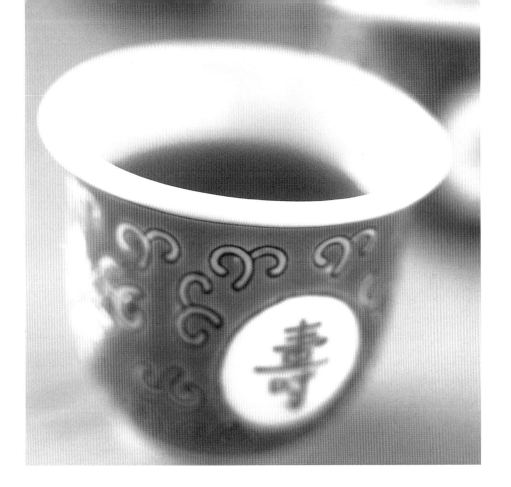

Pycnogenol – Derived from the extract of pine tree bark.

Polyphenols – Include flavonoids, or catechins, and appear to be powerful antioxidants. Certain flavonoids, including quercetin, have been shown to help prevent blood clots, and have anti-inflammatory properties.

Tocopherol – More commonly referred to as vitamin E, this oil-soluble antioxidant is used as an emollient and moisturizer by drawing water content from the dermis to the epidermis.

plant sources

Phytochemicals or plant chemicals have had a major impact on anti-ageing skin care. They may be the next antidote to maturing and withering.

Phytoestrogens

Phytoestrogens, called isoflavones, mimic the effects of the female hormone, oestrogen. Important phytoestrogens are genistein, daidzein, enterolactone and equol. These compounds may improve cholesterol, prevent bone loss and suppress enzymes that stimulate breast cancer. Newer wrinkle creams contain plant hormones, like wild yam extract - a plant source for progesterone, soya - a plant source for oestrogen, and melatonin - an antioxidant hormone that naturally triggers the sleep cycle. Milk thistle belongs to the same family as daisies and artichokes and is commonly taken for its anti-tumour properties. Soya Isoflavones may be helpful in preventing breast cancer, battling hot flushes and reducing the risk of heart disease. Chemically, they mimic the effect of oestrogen on the skin, which creeps away as the years fly by, causing dryness and loss of elasticity. Using hormones on your face works to keep skin hydrated, firm and toned.

Saponins

Saponins are forms of carbohydrates that neutralize enzymes in the intestines that may cause cancer. They may also boost the immune system and promote wound healing.

Capsaicin

Capsaicin seems to reduce levels of substance P, a compound that contributes to inflammation and the delivery of pain impulses from the central nervous system. It is found in hot red chilli peppers.

Enzymes

'N6-Furfuryladenine' the chemical name for a plant growth factor that has been compared to retinoids for its effect on the skin, is known to plump up the leaves of plants by causing the surface layer to retain water. Unlike traditional moisturizers that temporarily add moisture to soften the skin's texture, this enzyme enhances cell turnover. It is non-irritating so anyone can use it and is available in both a lotion and cream formula. This enzyme has the flexibility of being incorporated into a regime of AHAs, Retinol or Vitamin C, or used as an alternative, and is especially kind to recently peeled or lifted skin. Papain, an enzyme found in papaya, is also helpful in sloughing off dead skin cells.

Squalene

With extracts, essences and oils from olives being poured into luscious skin care formulas, this little Mediterranean fruit gets top billing. Olives are rich in Squalene, which can stimulate cells and enliven dry skin. Squalene belongs to the family of phytochemicals called sterols. The leaves are a source of Oleuropein; an antioxidant that destroys free radicals, the oil is rich in fatty acids and glycerides for hydration and the tree bark is a great natural exfoliant.

peel me a grape

Superficial peels basically accomplish three key things: exfoliation, moisturization and thickening the dermis. Any acid can be made to penetrate the skin lightly or deeply.

Used with active skin care, superficial peels or microdermabrasion speed up the process of exfoliation. This approach works best for modest sun damage, early wrinkling or just plain dull looking skin. Peels also work for pre-cancerous actinic keratoses (see page 23), hyperpigmentation and acne scarring. Full-face chemical peels remove an entire layer of skin at once.

Low concentrations of acid produce a superficial peel; high doses are used for deeper exfoliations. The basic principle is: the deeper the peel the better the result, the worse you look immediately afterwards and the longer it takes to heal. The other critical variable is the person who is doing the peeling and no peels are entirely idiot-proof. The word 'peel' is an umbrella term used to cover a wide range of treatments starting at the level of a mild glycolic wash from the chemist, all the way up to carbon dioxide laser resurfacing. Find out what acid is being applied and educate yourself about the various factors that affect the peel result; depth, concentration, how it is neutralized, length of time it is on the skin and so on. Peels can be adapted to various levels depending on your needs. Apart from a basic skin classification (light to dark and tendency to burn or tan), the other factors in deciding to have a superficial peel or a deeper version are lifestyle related. One good slough deserves another. Micro-

Microdermabraders are popular peel alternatives and peel boosters. Having a light microdermabrasion treatment, followed by an enzyme or acid peel, allows the solution to penetrate deeper.

The deep

Trichloracetic acid (TCA) peels (Obagi® and other brands) can penetrate deeper into the skin and remove the outer layers. These peels are thought to reconstitute the lower collagen and elastin layers of the skin. There is moderate swelling of the treated areas for about a week, and scabbing will occur. Deeper peels with more concentrated solutions may take up to 2 weeks to heal. TCA peels are good for fine wrinkles, mild scarring, age spots and to counteract sun damage and uneven pigmentation. Phenol peels and Croton Oil peels are experiencing a resurgence, and newer formulas are more buffered with less chance of skin whitening.

Any skin type is a candidate for some form of peeling, but the darker your skin, the fewer safe peeling options you have. The deeper the peel, the greater the risk of it having a bleaching or whitening effect (hyperpigmentation), a line of demarcation or temporary and even permanent scarring.

WARNING: DO NOT have any peel if you are taking RoAccutane (Accutane), or if you have Herpes Simplex or other open lesions. If you have a history of cold sores, ask your doctor for an anti-viral if having a peel or lasering around the mouth.

back to the future

Medical science is getting closer and closer to conquering ageing. The fountain of youth may come in the form of a hormone.

Growth hormones

Human Growth Hormone (HGH), produced in the body by the pituitary gland, is plentiful during childhood and adolescence, but its levels decrease dramatically as we age. HGH is credited with rejuvenating every cell in the body, adding 30 years to your life, bringing organs back to health, having you remember things you might rather forget and making studs out of grumpy old men. It should come as no surprise that HGH has taken off among celebs as the newest nectar of the Gods. At the heart of anti-ageing medicine lie injections of HGH, first used by athletes to build up muscle. Growth hormone is produced and secreted in pulses by the pituitary gland that move throughout the body affecting tissues, bones and muscles. Doctors began prescribing it for children in need of a growth boost, and later to treat wasting (loss of weight and strength) in AIDS patients.

Before you consider HGH therapy, be prepared to have every body function put under a microscope, literally. A comprehensive evaluation of nutritional, metabolic and hormonal levels, and vision screenings, bone-density scans, treadmill stress tests and brain assessments are done. The goal is to revert the body back to its healthiest state - around age 30. After 30, things measurably start to decline. To work, it has to be pharmaceutical grade growth hormone, not the new generation of products sold via the Internet and in health stores as dietary supplements, oral sprays and powders. The latter are usually formulations of amino acids that allegedly trigger the release of HGH in the body.

Research now suggests that topical growth factors may help reverse the signs of ageing in skin. Growth factors work differently to vitamins A and C to stimulate collagen. The trick is to get growth factors, which are large proteins, to penetrate the dermis. This is currently being studied. Nouricel-MD®, a solution containing key growth factors cited for skin rejuvenation, is at the forefront of this new technology.

Sex hormones

The use of sex hormones to reverse wrinkles is being touted as one of the next frontiers in anti-ageing medicine. Hormones naturally found in the body include: oestrogen, progesterone, DHEA (dehydroepiandrosterone), androstenedione and testosterone. As we age, the production of hormones decreases progressively and everything dries out. Compounded hormones and DHEA creams could be the wave of the future, and studies have shown positive effects on ageing skin.

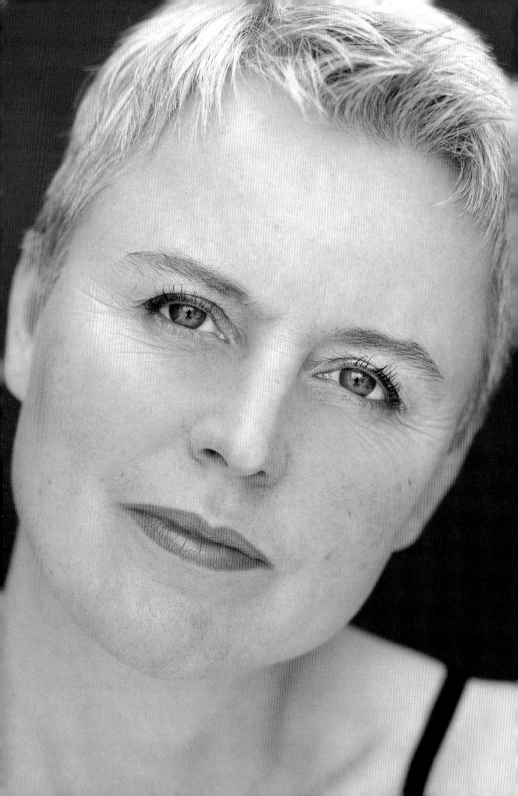

ZAPPING THEM

ZAPPING THEM

Topical products can only do so much to improve the appearance of the skin. If you want to see more dramatic improvements, you have to look to deeper remedies, the kind of treatments performed by cosmetic surgeons, dermatologists and registered nurses. Today there is a wide choice of facial rejuvenation techniques, making it possible to tailor therapies to your exact needs. A variety of methods are used to remove the topmost layers of the skin, revealing clear, unblemished skin below. These are called skin resurfacing.

Resurfacing with lasers has traditionally involved ablative procedures that necessitated long recovery procedures and left patients red-faced for weeks or months. Although these techniques work, they are riskier and messier than many of us are willing to put up with. The newer non-ablative techniques can deliver collagen remodelling that works on your wrinkles in a kinder, gentler way.

laser resurfacing

Laser resurfacing can remove wrinkles and red veins, lighten discolourations and age spots and smooth scars, as well as stimulate fibroblasts to increase collagen production.

A laser is a high-energy beam of light that selectively directs its energy into the tissue. It works like a high-tech scalpel that allows the doctor greater control and finesse. The laser (Light Amplification by the Stimulated Emission of Radiation) is a 'light pump'. It applies the principles of radiation physics to narrowly segregate light of a selected wavelength and 'pump' the light radiation to high intensity. The beams are targeted to a specific spot and are varied in intensity and in the duration of emitted pulses depending on their mission. Lasers and light sources are the modern way to pulverize wrinkles and extract redness from the skin. They have virtually left many older techniques in the dust.

Resurfacing with a laser should be performed in a doctor's surgery, either by a doctor or a trained nurse under medical supervision. It can be done under local anaesthetic with or without intravenous sedation, or a topical anaesthetic cream or spray can be used for more superficial procedures. Depending on the extent of the treatment, the work can take anywhere from a few minutes to more than an hour. The laser is passed over parts of the face, neck, chest or hands, and evaporates the surface layers of the targeted areas of skin. A new layer of pink skin is revealed.

Generally, the more passes with the laser and the deeper the setting, the more extensive the treatment and longer the recovery.

The newest lasers penetrate through to the layers beneath to boost collagen production, which gives the skin a plumper, tighter appearance. Treatments improve skin texture and tone by stimulating new collagen in the skin to smooth it out from underneath the surface. These treatments do not destroy outer tissue as they work their way down to stimulate collagen growth in the dermis, so they are safe to use on most skin types. Your doctor will be able to advise you. The process is gradual and the softening of wrinkles occurs over time. You will need multiple treatment sessions in order to see results and the improvement is much less dramatic. No pain, no gain. Don't expect to be wrinkle-free at the end of one course. The advantage is zero recovery time and you won't turn scarlet for months.

TOP TIP:
Laser treatments should be done under the supervision of a medical doctor who is properly trained in laser surgery. All lasers can be dangerous in the wrong hands.

waves of the future

Lasers are classified in two categories; ablative, which are reserved for deeper wrinkles and creases, and non-ablative, which improve the skin's quality, texture and tone.

Ablative lasers

Ablative laser technology causes a burn which 'ablates' or removes the upper layers of skin to promote the growth of pink new skin underneath. These high-tech tools focus laser energy on damaged surface layers of skin and vaporize them, which allows a fresh layer to emerge and stimulates fibroblasts. Because of the laser beam's precision, the doctor can make several passes over areas that require extra attention without harm to adjacent skin. The two most frequently used deeper lasers for skin resurfacing are carbon dioxide CO_2 and Erbium:YAG.

Non-ablative lasers

Non-ablative laser and light sources are proving to be a good gentle alternative for the laser phobic. The newcomers in the rapidly changing laser universe work by stimulating new collagen in the dermis, called subsurface remodelling. They essentially treat wrinkles from the inside out, rather than removing them from the outside. The laser's heat bypasses the epidermis and encourages fibroblast production, thickening the underlying collagen structure. The process of softening wrinkles continues over time as the rejuvenated skin fibres reach the surface. Non-exfoliating rejuvenating lasers are ideal for younger women who want to prevent, postpone or maintain more invasive treatments. Procedures are repeated every 4 to 6 weeks over a 6-month period to maximize new collagen formation, and are performed on an area larger than that you want to improve; for example, lower eyelids would include the upper cheeks in order to get a progressive tightening. Since non-ablative lasers have a very long wavelength, they are safe for most skin types. This technology is faster than the ablative laser, recovery is shorter, there is less risk of pigment changes and little or no discomfort. Although non-ablative lasers won't erase wrinkles and brown spots to the same degree as their ablative cousins, they are perfect for maintenance after deeper resurfacing, or as part of a maintenance programme in combination with skin care and microdermabrasion treatments. This new laser generation is growing and we will see more variations on this technology in the near future.

laser toning

Although non-invasive resurfacing offers a lower degree of collagen remodelling than more invasive approaches do, lunchtime treatments are definitely what women want.

Non-ablative systems deliver controlled energy to the skin in slightly different ways, but their mission is basically the same. The 'N-Lite' Laser Collagen Replenishment System, FDA-cleared for the reduction of wrinkles around the eyes, uses a specific frequency of yellow laser light to gently stimulate growth of your body's own collagen layer. As new collagen forms, it begins to fill in the wrinkles, therefore reducing surface lines. Protective goggles are worn during the treatment which takes 15 minutes, and most women experience a mild tingling or slight redness, but can wear make-up right away. Any visible reduction in wrinkles requires at least 30 days to appear and may continue to improve for up to 90 days. The newly formed collagen will then age at the normal rate and the procedure is repeated for maintenance as needed.

The sister treatments to the Pulsed Dye laser technology, like the 'N-Lite' System, are called 'near infrared wavelengths', ND:Yag lasers. This technology, like the CoolTouch®, heats the water in the upper dermis to create a thermal wound using a cooling cryogen spray to protect the epidermis from damage. The body's response is to produce new collagen.

Intense pulsed light sources work by creating a wound in the small blood vessels in the dermis that causes collagen and vessels under the top layer to constrict. These treatments are done in a series of 3-week intervals. There may be some minor discomfort, often described as similar to a rubber band snapping against the skin. A topical cream can be applied before treatment and there will be some redness and swelling that may last for 1–5 days. The visible reduction of fine lines and wrinkles occurs gradually over the next few weeks or months. This treatment is good for fine lines – particularly around the eyes and mouth, shallow acne scars, age spots, spider veins, rosacea, sun damage, large pores and dark circles around the eyes. It can also be used to treat areas on the neck, arms, chest and hands.

Pure light treatments are a non-laser alternative for reducing fine lines and wrinkles. Pure light treatments like Enlighten® can stimulate the body's natural tissue-remodelling process to improve skin smoothness. The light is painless and safe, and can be used for all skin types. Multiple treatments will be needed to see results, and a top up session is recommended every 3 months after the initial treatment course to maintain results.

BEAUTY BYTES:
To find out more about 'N-Lite', log on to
www.wrinklereduction.com

high beams

Ablative laser resurfacing is not a casual undertaking. Doctors love the effects of Carbon Dioxide laser treatments, but the downside is the prolonged healing and redness.

Carbon dioxide

Pulsed carbon dioxide laser skin resurfacing is the gold standard for removing thin layers of skin with minimal heat damage. The laser energy is delivered to the skin at the point where superficial tissue is vaporized and destroyed and dermal damage causes collagen remodelling and skin contraction. CO_2 lasers can reach deeper wrinkles, but this is a serious treatment with a long recovery period. CO_2 is still considered the workhorse of lasers because of its dramatic results on deeper wrinkles, scarring and sun damage. Typically, you will be required to apply an occlusive ointment that water cannot penetrate, for 7–10 days. The epidermis regenerates at that point, but the skin takes several weeks, up to 3 months, to return to normal. The fairer your skin, the longer you will stay pink. CO_2 lasers are not recommended for darker complexions because they can alter the pigment in the skin, leaving it darker or lighter.

BEAUTY BYTES:

To find out more about lasers, visit
www.asds-net.org, www.aslms.org
and www.surgery.org

Erbium:YAG

Erbium:YAG technology emits energy in the mid-infrared invisible light spectrum and is considered a second cousin to CO_2. Unlike CO_2 lasers, Er:YAGs produce little thermal effect. They target the skin itself and the wavelengths are absorbed by the water. Since most of our cells are predominantly water, they get absorbed by the first cells they touch. The heat effects of the laser are scattered so that thin layers of tissue can be removed with precision while minimizing damage to surrounding skin. Erbium is used for sculpting deeper lines that remain after CO_2 resurfacing, and for fine lines, mild sun damage and superficial scars. Treatment can be repeated if needed. Longer pulsed Erbium lasers deliver results that fall somewhere between CO_2 and traditional Erbium. They provide more wrinkle relief than Erbium alone, with less risk of scarring than the CO_2. Lighter ablative models, like the variable-pulsed Erbium, are also popular because they are safer for darker skin types. Combining Erbium with CO_2 can produce better results and speed up the long healing process that has turned many of us off lasers. Deeper lasers are being used more superficially so that you can look good after a week and the pinkness fades quickly. These treatments are good for mild to moderate skin damage.

laser trends

Future lasers will be developed to offer the same degree of improvement as ablative systems, without the effects and down time.

The main challenges faced by lasers focus on risks versus benefits, and their safety when used on darker skin types. The darker the skin colour, the more risk of lightening, darkening or scarring from resurfacing treatments. If you have freckles on parts of your face, deeper laser resurfacing performed on one regional area like around the mouth, the lower eyelid area, or the forehead instead of the full face, may leave you with an uneven appearance. Although the lighter lasers are not able to eradicate wrinkles and brown spots as well, they are more appealing to women who are unwilling or unable to put up with a long recovery. Non-ablative techniques are good for anyone who can't take the time out for deeper procedures, or who can't commit to staying out of the sun. For extensive sun damage, different wavelengths are required.

Another technology is electrosurgical resurfacing using coblation, a micro-electrical radio frequency. Coblation delivers a pulse of energy instead of heat, to the surface of the skin. It seals blood vessels as it removes tissue and promotes skin tightening as a laser would, but by a dramatically cooler process. Electrosurgical resurfacing is good for most

TOP TIP:

As with any series or course, microdermabrasions and non-ablative laser treatments are best done one at a time and repeated as needed. If after a few treatments you don't see any improvement, you can assume it's not going to work as you expected and switch to another method so you are not locked in.

skin types, and the swelling and redness usually clears in 2–4 weeks. It can be used to improve superficial to moderate skin damage and is generally a less expensive alternative with slightly faster healing than some lasers, but the benefits may not last as long.

The aftermath

The big drawback of ablative lasers is the 7–14 days of postoperative care. After the skin has been treated, it is covered with either a thin film of ointment or cream, or a light synthetic breathable dressing to protect the new skin as it heals. Expect some redness, oozing, swelling, itching and discomfort. It is critical that you follow your doctor's instructions on the proper aftercare, to the letter. Applying ice packs can reduce swelling and relieve discomfort for the first 48 hours, but you will be instructed not to get the area wet. You may have to drink through a straw after treatments around the mouth area. Absolutely NO sun exposure will be allowed, preferably forever, or at least 6–8 weeks.

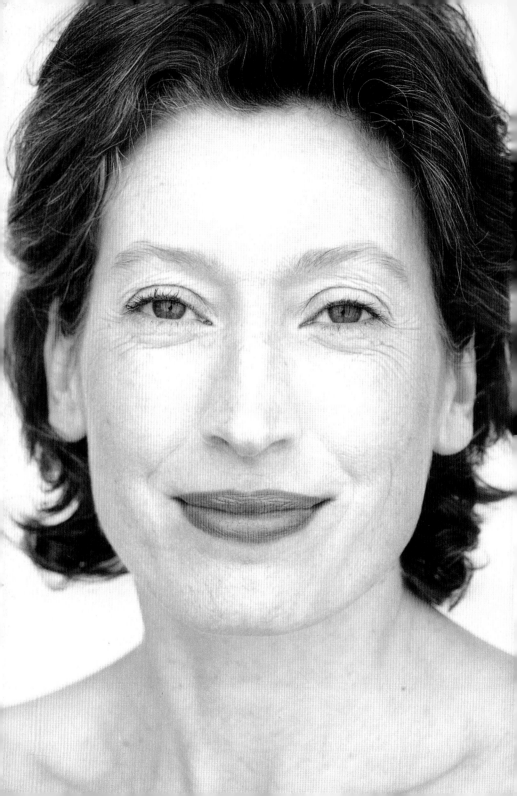

NEEDLE POINTS

There comes a point in every woman's life when all the creams, peels and lasers together aren't enough to plump up lines, creases and canyons. That's the time to look to wrinkle fillers. It doesn't mean you should stop all your other treatments. Fillers are just another method to add to your maintenance programme. All of the minimally invasive treatments described in this book compliment each other. Think of wrinkle remedies like a menu in a Chinese restaurant. Take a bit from each column to put together your perfect rejuvenation menu, and add to it as the lines get deeper. The best method is an integrated approach that may begin with one or a combination of para-surgical treatments. It's never too early to start formulating a plan for your wrinkle future.

Botulinum Toxin has become the cornerstone of any anti-ageing programme for the face. No other single product has revolutionized cosmetic medicine so much in such a relatively short time. According to The American Society for Aesthetic Plastic Surgery, in 2000, 1.6 million BOTOX® injections were performed. It is rare to find any BOTOX® candidate who hasn't been positively thrilled with the results. It also gives the best value for money.

freezing them

BOTOX® has proven to be a little poison with unlimited health and beauty potential. A few precious drops can manage everything from frown lines, worry lines, upper lip creases and neck cords, to excessive sweating and migraines.

There are various strains of Botulinum Toxin. Type A is the most potent.

Type A

Botulinum Toxin Type A purified neurotoxin complex has been used since 1980 to treat muscle disorders, such as lazy eye, eye ticks and uncontrolled blinking. Pioneered by an ophthalmologist in 1987, its wide range of cosmetic uses have made it a mainstay in the cosmetic surgeon's arsenal of weapons for mass destruction of facial wrinkles. It had been considered an 'off-label' use of an FDA-approved drug until it received approval for cosmetic use in Canada and most recently, from the last frontier, the US Food and Drug Administration (FDA). In 2001, Botulinum Toxin Type A was approved in the UK for use in controlling excessive sweating in the underarm, called 'hyperhydrosis'. With small injections of toxin directly into the underarm skin, or on the palms of the hand or soles of the foot, the sweat glands become paralyzed.

Type B

Botulinum Toxin Type B has been introduced more recently, marketed under the name MYOBLOC™ in the US and NEUROBLOC™ in the EC. It is approved for use in the treatment of cervical dystonia, a neurological disorder, and not yet approved for cosmetic uses. This form comes as a pre-made liquid that does not require a diluting agent, and is typically preserved in normal saline. Compared with Type A, it has a longer shelf life of up to 2 years and works slightly faster but is also slightly more painful when injected. Clinical studies are underway to determine the most effective dosages for this latest form.

Botulinum Toxin Type A is available under the trade name BOTOX®, which is manufactured by Allergan Inc, and Dysport®, manufactured by Ipsen Ltd. Type B can be found under the name MYOBLOC™ or NEUROBLOC™. They are made by Elan Pharmaceuticals and Elan Corp, respectively.

beauty of BOTOX®

After getting over the idea of having poison injected into their faces, most women get hooked. Just one treatment brings a noticeable improvement and softening of facial lines.

There is literally no age that is too soon to start, and women in their late 20s and 30s are into Botulinum Toxin in a big way, as the foundation of an early battle against ageing. Unlike fillers that temporarily plump up creases but don't really prevent them from getting deeper or stop new ones from forming, it slows down the formation of new facial lines. Combining Botulinum Toxin to stop new lines from forming, with treatments for the lines already there, is the best way to maintain a lineless look.

New uses are discovered frequently, as doctors are becoming more experimental with its potent effects.

Where it works

vertical lines between the brows

lines at the bridge of the nose

crow's-feet or squint lines

horizontal forehead lines

muscle bands on the neck

under eyelid creases

décolleté lines

chin crease

drooping corners of the mouth

upper lip lines

How it works

The toxin acts on the junctions between nerves and muscles, preventing the release of a chemical messenger called acetylcholine from the nerve endings. Tiny amounts are injected into a specific facial muscle so only the targeted impulse of that muscle will be blocked, causing a local relaxation. It acts as a muscle blockade to immobilize the underlying cause of the unwanted lines – muscle contractions – and prevent 'wrinkly' expressions. Since the muscle can no longer make the offending facial expression, the lines gradually smooth out from disuse and new creases are prevented from forming. Other muscles that are not treated are not affected, so a natural look and expressions are maintained. It may not be as effective on lines that are not entirely caused by the action of a muscle, e.g. the nasal labial folds that are formed by a combination of muscle action and the weight of sagging skin. Some areas are less suited to this procedure because the muscles are needed for expression and important functions like eating, kissing and opening the eyes. The goal is not to knock out every muscle twinge – it is a softening of dynamic facial lines that won't necessarily betray your wrinkle reducing secret.

frozen assets

- Have your first treatment with someone who comes highly recommended and has a lot of experience, so that in future you will know what is acceptable.

- Start small with one area, typically the lines between the brows or crow's-feet. Once you see the results, you can decide to have more areas worked on at your next treatment.

- If you are squeamish about needles, ask your doctor for a topical anaesthetic cream .

- To relieve the discomfort of the injections, apply an ice pack before and after treatment .

- If your treatment didn't work, you may have been given an overly diluted solution and need more, or it could have been injected into the wrong spot. It is exceedingly rare to be resistant to it.

- Take along a concealer to cover needle marks or tiny bruises right after treatment, so you will be happy to be seen in public.

- Plan your day around having your treatment – you should remain upright for 3–4 hours afterwards.

- It is possible to get a slight headache after the first few sessions. This will usually go away within a couple of days.

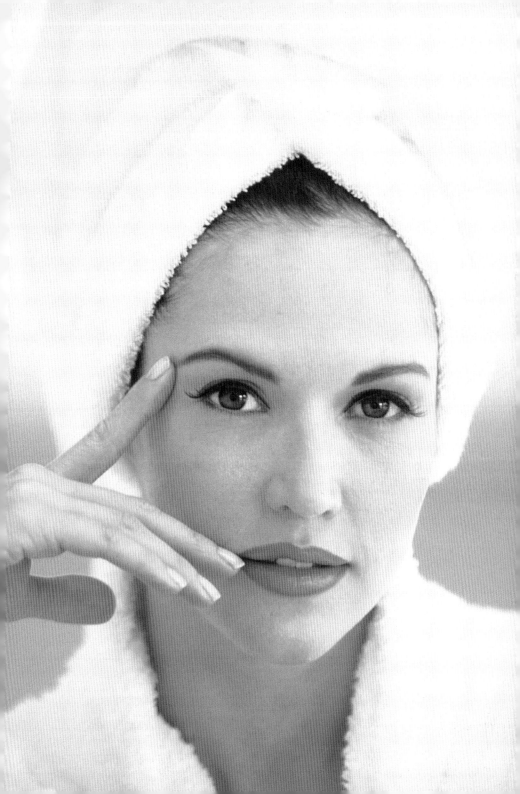

BOTOX® budgeting

Botulinum Toxin takes effect 3 to 7 days after treatment. The improvement generally lasts for 3 to 6 months, before the effect gradually fades and muscle action returns.

Doctors set their fees by the area, by the treatment, or based on how much material they inject. Each area to be treated is considered a zone; for example, the crow's-feet on both sides of your face would be considered one zone; horizontal forehead lines constitute another zone; the frown lines between your eyebrows would be another zone. Each zone is usually priced separately, but most doctors discount the fee for the second and third areas. If the price for one zone is £250, having a second area done at the same time may cost you only an additional £200. The most common combination of areas to have done in one go is: glabellar, forehead and crow's-feet. The muscle bands of the neck may be priced higher than the glabellar because more toxin is often required to get the job done. If you decide to do a little more for this line or that because he is there already, don't be surprised to be charged an additional amount. Ask ahead of time what the fee will be for your treatment so you are prepared.

A single treatment will normally be sustained for approximately three months, with some variation. In areas where there are two sides to be injected, as in the forehead or crow's-feet, the toxin may fade unevenly and the lines on one side return more than the lines on the other. When you begin to notice a gradual fading of its effects, you should have your next treatment. Don't wait until all of it has worn off – keep up with your treatments. When you are able to contract your facial muscles, go back for a touch-up. If you stay on top of it, you will look consistently unlined all the time. If you wait six months between treatments, until all or most of it has worn off, it will be a telltale sign that you are a BOTOX® user since you will look different at the tail end of your treatment to just after it. Basically, you can expect to have a treatment 3–4 times a year. Beware of discounted BOTOX® – you may be paying less because you are getting less. Some doctors over dilute Botulinum Toxin Type A or keep it around for too long so it loses its potency, so they can stretch more treatments out of a vial. The result is that your wrinkles won't stay frozen as well or for as long. Instead of getting a good result for 4 months, it may only last for 2, and there goes your savings!

Brilliant BOTOX®

Very little can go wrong with Botulinum Toxin, and the good news is that if it does, it is temporary. The only complications you can have are an occasional eyelid droop, an asymmetry or a crooked mouth. Side effects are rarely serious and always temporary, and even if you don't like the results, they are guaranteed to go away as the toxin wears off. The problems are purely about technique and some injectors are just simply better than others. The minimum amount to be effective, no more and no less, is what is recommended. If you're worried about safety, ask your doctor whether he injects himself, his wife, or his staff, all of which are common.

filling station

For decades, wrinkles have been filled with human-derived tissues, most specifically fat. Today, natural and synthetic fillers are available and new ones keep popping up.

The plumping of lines using our own tissue is a popular treatment. Fat is taken from buttocks, hips or thighs and re-injected into the necessary areas. The process involves three phases: harvesting, storing for future use and injecting. It takes longer to perform than injecting an off-the-shelf filler. Doctors rarely agree on the best technique. Variables include how the fat is extracted, where it is injected, how deeply and how much. It isn't a one time event. As your own tissue is used, you won't be allergic to it. Fat grafting is performed under a local anaesthetic and can take from 30 minutes to a few hours, depending on the extent of the work. Much of the face is suitable for transplants – the lips, nasal labial folds and cheek hollows are among the most common. Expect postop swelling and bruising to last for up to a week.

Fat transfer has become the first choice for volume filling. Like all injectables, fat lasts better in static lines than in mobile areas such as around the mouth. It is widely accepted as a stand alone procedure, or in combination with cosmetic facial surgery, BOTOX® and resurfacing.

Other fillers can be fashioned from materials from tissue banks. or your own fascia, skin, muscle and cartilage. Studies are underway to use human foreskin as a wrinkle filler. Isolagen™ is a process that enables you to grow your own collagen cells. Commercially available forms include Fascialata (Fascian®) and Dermal Tissue (Cymetra®, AlloDerm®).

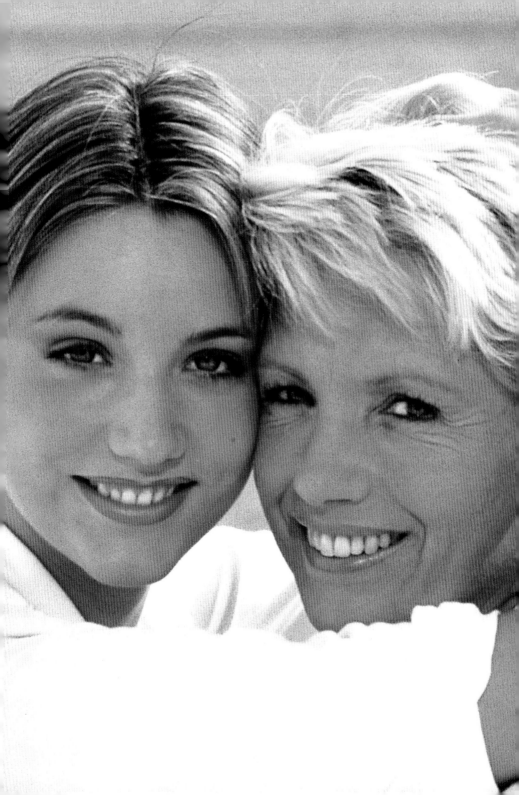

between the lines

Wrinkle fillers turn up on the market constantly, but it takes time to establish the long-term safety of new formulas. Approval varies from country to country.

New fillers are always under clinical investigation, and products with a high incidence of complications have difficulty getting approval in America. In Europe, they must be approved with an EC Mark. In the US, they fall under the domain of the FDA, which has more stringent requirements. Since the advent of BOTOX®, fillers have been used less frequently for the forehead and around the eyes. If the creases between the brows are very deep, a filler could be used in addition, but BOTOX® is usually done first.

Resorbable

Resorbable fillers are made from natural or synthetic materials that are broken down and resorbed by the body. They are temporary and will need to be re-injected, typically in 3–9 months. You can have other fillers injected into the same area later on. Of these, hyaluronic acid is gaining recognition as the most promising.

Non-resorbable

This class of fillers has synthetic components that don't get broken down by the body. They are permanent and cannot be removed. The ageing process continues, so even if your lines are injected with a permanent filler, you will need additional treatments down the road.

Wrinkle fillers

Type	Brand Name
Resorbable	
Bovine collagen (cow)	Zyplast®, Zyderm®
Bovine collagen with PMMA particles	ArteColl®
Bovine collagen	Resoplast®
Hyaluronic acid gel (bacteria based – non-animal)	Restylane®, Restylane Fine
Hyaluronic acid gel (from poultry)	Hylaform®, Hylaform Plus®, Hylaform Fine®
Hyaluronic acid gel with PMMA particles	Dermalive®
Polylactic acid	NewFill®
Polyacrilamide copolymer gel	Outline®
Acrylic hydrogel	Dermadeep®
Non-resorbable	
Injectable liquid silicone	Adatosil 5000®, Silikon 1000®
Methacrylate microspheres	Meta-crill®, Arteplast®
Polyacrylamide gel	Aquamid®

This is a partial list, including just the fillers used most commonly in various parts of the world. Trade names vary depending on the country or region.

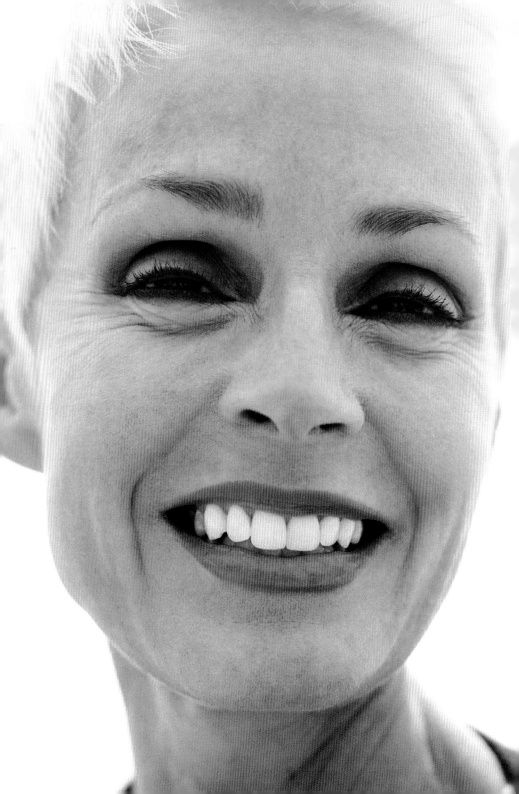

dos and don'ts for fillers

- **DO** tell your doctor of any history of bleeding and blood clots before you have a treatment.

- **DON'T** take aspirin or vitamin E supplements for 1 to 2 weeks before treatment.

- **DO** use a vitamin K cream before and after treatment to minimize bruising.

- **DO** apply ice compresses immediately following treatment to minimize swelling.

- **DON'T** schedule your beauty shots for the week of your period because you are more sensitive or prone to bruising.

- **DON'T** have any fillers or treatments while pregnant ot breastfeeding.

filler prep

New wrinkle fillers turn up on the market constantly, but it takes time to establish the long-term safety of newly released formulas.

The newest product may not always be the best available and doctors need time to determine the advantages and/or disadvantages of any new product in comparison to existing fillers on the market. The results may look fine right now, but you'll want to know that as you age and your skin thins, you won't see or feel lumps and bumps hardening due to the use of synthetic particles. The safest wrinkle filler treatments are generally those that have the longest and best track record, meaning more people have had treatments successfully. Some women won't accept the idea of having an unknown material injected into their faces. Synthetic fillers or fillers that contain synthetic particles are usually designed to last longer than natural ones, but are more risky. If you are skeptical about the origins of any wrinkle treatment, stick with your own fat because you definitely know where that comes from.

ONLY Medical Doctors and Registered Nurses (usually under the supervision of a Medical Doctor) are properly trained to administer wrinkle fillers. Be careful about using a technician whose qualifications you are not sure of. Keep records of what treatment you had and when you had it.

TOP TIP:
Never be a guinea pig for a brand new wrinkle filler treatment. Wait until it has been used for 3-5 years before having it used on you.

questionnaire

Questions to ask your doctor

- What is the source of the material?

- Is it natural or synthetic?

- What is the name of the manufacturer and where are they located? (Ask to see a product brochure.)

- How long has the filler been on the market?

- What kinds of clinical studies have been carried out on the filler?

- Is it FDA-approved or does it have the EC mark?

- How long has the doctor/nurse been using it?

- What are the possible side effects?

- Do I need a skin test before treatment?

- Could I be allergic to the filler?

- What does a reaction look like and how long does it last?

- What can be done if I have a reaction to it?

- What are the risks?

- How many treatments will I need and how often?

- How much will each treatment cost?

- If it doesn't look right, what can be done to remove it?

- Can I still have other fillers later on?

lighten up

When you're young, they are called freckles. By your 40s, they are referred to as 'age' or 'liver spots'. Hyperpigmentation or solar lentigenes can ruin your creamy complexion.

Age spots don't discriminate. They attack almost any part of the body that has been chronically exposed to the sun's harmful rays. Skin lighteners bleach out dark or brown spots on the skin. Hydroquinone and Kojic acid are the two most common formulas. For best results, prescription-strength bleaching agents are recommended. Over-the-counter cosmetics won't be very effective because the levels of key ingredients aren't high enough to produce visible results. If you follow a prescription bleaching regime religiously, you could see real improvement in as little as 4–6 weeks. Tyrosinase inhibitors help to block melanin production, which causes pigmentation of the skin.

Kojic acid – is an antibacterial agent and tyrosinase inhibitor. It is very effective at lightening hyperpigmentation without causing irritation as seen with the use of hydroquinone, so is suitable for hydroquinone-allergic patients. It is a water-soluble antibiotic produced by the fermentation of a mushroom, *fungi aspergillis.*

Arbutin – is found in bearberry extract and acts as a potent tyrosinase inhibitor to assist in lightening areas of hyperpigmentation.

Azelaic acid – is an effective tyrosinase inhibitor that helps to lighten hyperpigmentation.

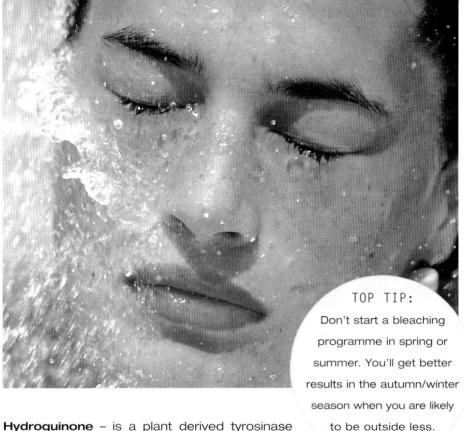

TOP TIP:

Don't start a bleaching programme in spring or summer. You'll get better results in the autumn/winter season when you are likely to be outside less.

Hydroquinone – is a plant derived tyrosinase inhibitor, hydroquinone can also be synthetically derived from phenol. It helps to inhibit melanin activity in the skin and lighten existing pigmentation. In high percentages, it is known to cause irritation and inflammation. Its use is banned in Japan and Australia.

Kligman's Formula – was developed by retinoid expert, Albert Kligman MD. This is a compound that contains tretinoin, hydroquinone and a mild steroid to cut down on irritation. It can be formulated by a pharmacist under the direction of your doctor.

Vitamin C – is not a tyrosinase inhibitor but a natural skin lightener, anti-inflammatory and skin strengthener/tightener. Limiting inflammation will help to inhibit melanocyte activity while Vitamin C's lightening capabilities can even out the complexion.

SUMMING IT UP

In theory, we could all prevent our skin from wrinkling. If you could protect your face from the sun all the time, it would remain relatively young looking and wrinkle-free into old age. In the past, however, this has not tended to happen, particularly because people have not understood the cause of photoageing. When people start hinting that it's time to take a new approach to your beauty maintenance routine, or the mirror betrays your age, today's extensive menu of non-surgical, minimally-invasive treatments have something for everyone, even for the scalpel-shy.

There are numerous treatments for wrinkles and lines – starting with topical tretinoin (Retin A®) and alphahydroxy acids and superficial peels and microdermabrasion that work similarly by stripping away the top layers of skin. Lines can be filled in by injecting a substance like fat or hyaluronic acid gel. The action of muscles causing certain lines can be weakened by using botulinum toxin. Resurfacing can be accomplished with deeper peeling or laser resurfacing. Generally, more aggressive, invasive procedures produce faster, more dramatic results but these are more costly, riskier and involve longer recoveries. Choosing the best approach depends on your lifestyle and your goals.

Para-surgical solutions go far to bridge the gap between what you can get at a beauty salon and the cosmetic surgeon's operating theatre. The real benefits of these treatments are that they are simple, fast and affordable, with few side effects and they don't interfere with your schedule or leave you looking like you've had anything done. They won't produce miracles, but they go a long way to make you look revitalized and refreshed.

For the best results, throw in some homegrown treatments in between trips to a professional. For dehydrated, sun damaged skin, there's no time to waste. Skip the basics and go straight to enzymes and AHAs and start sloughing. For super sensitive skin, go lightly and stay scrub-phobic. Heat, steam, pressure and massage can aggravate delicate skin. Save the acids for later.

New technologies are emerging into the field of anti-ageing treatments as fast as dot coms these days. Advances among tools for diagnosis and treatment in medicine will eventually filter down into plastic surgery, dermatology and dentistry. These developments, coupled with the growing acceptance worldwide of the Internet as a source for health and medicine information, will revolutionize the speciality and reduce the barriers that many women are faced with when they think about doing something to their wrinkles and bags. The world has become a much smaller place and discoveries are shared at a much faster rate between specialists across countries and continents. The most exciting aspect of the field of aesthetic medicine is that it is constantly evolving and you never know what's coming next.

index

acknowledgments

Special thanks to my gorgeous girl Eden Claire for giving me a reason to write. My great appreciation goes to Alison Cathie and Jane O'Shea for having a vision, and to Lisa Pendreigh and Katie Ginn for making it work.

I also wish to thank the many doctors, surgeons and experts who kindly gave their time and shared their knowledge with me to help with my research. Tina Alster; Lena Andersson; Patrick Bowler; Frederic Brandt; Anita Cela; Dai Davies; Lisa Donofrio; Bryan Forley; Nellie Gauthier; Ellen Gendler; Roy Geronemus; Arielle Kauvar; Arnold Klein; Val Lambros; Albert Lefkovits; Elaine Linker, President, DDF Labs; Z. Paul Lorenc; Nicholas Lowe; Alan Matarasso; Seth Matarasso; Daniel Morello; Foad Nahai; Nicholas Percival; Laurie Polis; Patricia Wexler; Donald Wood-Smith.

picture credits

For more information on wrinkle rescues visit Wendy Lewis's website at www.wlbeauty.com or email your skin care queries to wlbeauty@aol.com.